Mediterranean Recipes for Busy People

An Amazing Collection of Super-Quick and Easy Recipes to Boost Your Metabolism and Improve Your Taste

Carl Ewing

Table of Contents

Salmon and Spinach Cups.. 5

Corn Salsa 7

Mushroom Snack 9

Black Beans and Coconut Spread 11

Chili and Fennel Bowls.......................................13

Sprouts Bites 15

Walnuts Snack 17

Radish Chips 19

Leeks Bowls 21

Creamy Leeks Dip..23

Peppers Cups 25

Coconut Avocado Spread 27

Lemon Corn Dip...29

Beans and Chia Power Bars..................................31

Apple Chips Mix 33

Yogurt Dip 35

Beet Bites..37

Pecans Bowls 39

Salmon Muffins..41

Squash Bites 43

Green Beans Snack Bowls....................................45

Broccoli and Shrimp Bars.....................................47

Pineapple and Basil Salsa.....................................49

Lemon Pork Chops 51

Lime Pork and Berries Mix....................................53

Cilantro Pork 55

Pepper Chops 57

Herbed Pork 59

Paprika Pork and Scallions 61

Cumin Pork Chops 63

Spiced Pork Mix 65

Pork and Asparagus 67

Pork and Black Beans 69

Peppercorn Pork Mix 71

Balsamic Oregano Pork 73

Sage Pork Mix 75

Pork Chops and Tomato Sauce 77

Pork Chops and Citrus Sauce 79

Allspice Pork 81

Pork with Mushrooms 83

Chili Cinnamon Pork Mix 85

Pork with Cabbage 87

Pork with Scallions and Cauliflower 89

Paprika Pork with Grapes 91

Pork with Kale 93

Balsamic Pork 95

Cumin Pork and Mango Mix 97

Pork and Pine Nuts Mix 99

Pork with Tomatoes and Endives 101

Pork and Shallots Pan 103

Mint Pork and Almonds 105

Pork and Zucchinis 107

Pork and Pinto Beans 109

Salmon and Spinach Cups

Prep time: 10 minutes I **Cooking time:** 0 minutes I
Servings: 6

Ingredients:

- 1 tablespoon avocado oil
- 1 tablespoon balsamic vinegar
- ½ teaspoon oregano, dried
- 1 cup smoked salmon, boneless, skinless and cubed
- 1 cup salsa
- 4 cups baby spinach

Directions:

1. In a bowl, combine the salmon with the salsa and the other ingredients, toss, divide into small cups and serve.

Nutrition facts per serving: calories 281, fat 14.4, fiber 7.4, carbs 18.7, protein 7.4

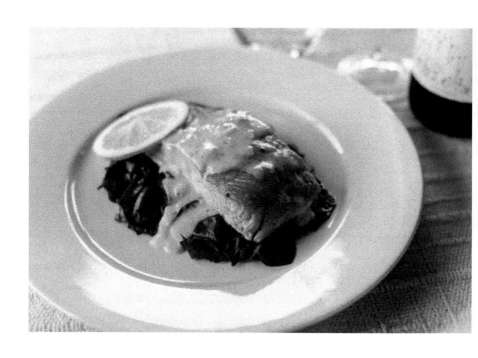

Corn Salsa

Prep time: 4 minutes I **Cooking time:** 0 minutes I

Servings: 4

Ingredients:

- 3 cups corn
- 2 cups tomatoes, cubed
- 2 green onions, chopped
- 2 tablespoons olive oil
- 1 red chili pepper, chopped
- ½ tablespoon chives, chopped

Directions:

1. In a salad bowl, combine the tomatoes with the corn and the other ingredients, toss and serve cold as a snack.

Nutrition facts per serving: calories 178, fat 8.6, fiber 4.5, carbs 25.9, protein 4.7

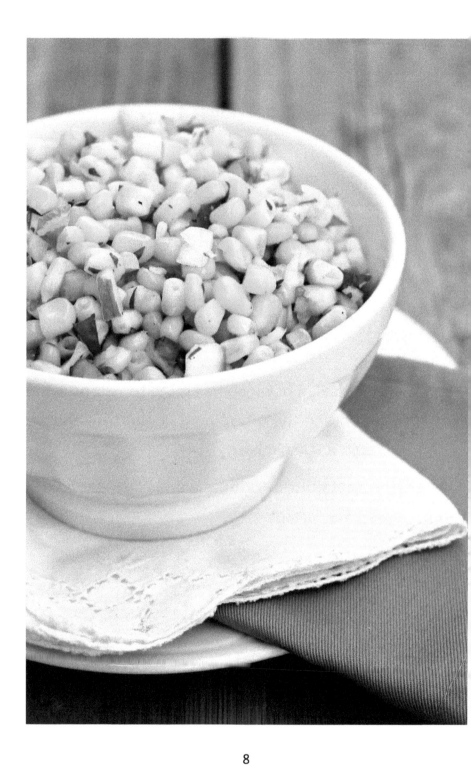

Mushroom Snack

Prep time: 10 minutes I **Cooking time:** 25 minutes I

Servings: 4

Ingredients:

- 1 pound small mushroom caps
- 2 tablespoons olive oil
- 1 tablespoon chives, chopped
- 1 tablespoon rosemary, chopped
- Black pepper to the taste

Directions:

1. Put the mushrooms in a roasting pan, add the oil and the rest of the ingredients, toss, bake at 400 degrees F for 25 minutes, divide into bowls and serve as a snack.

Nutrition facts per serving: calories 215, fat 12.3, fiber 6.7, carbs 15.3, protein 3.5

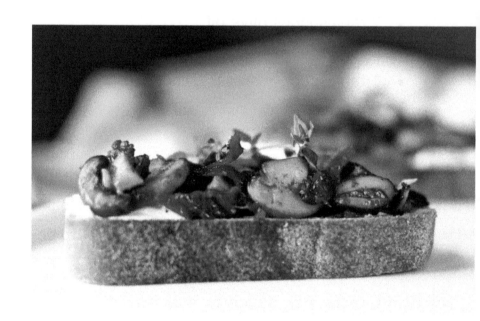

Black Beans and Coconut Spread

Prep time: 5 minutes I **Cooking time:** 0 minutes I

Servings: 4

Ingredients:

- ½ cup coconut cream
- 1 tablespoon olive oil
- 2 cups black beans, cooked
- 2 tablespoons green onions, chopped

Directions:

1. In a blender, combine the beans with the cream and the other ingredients, pulse well, divide into bowls and serve.

Nutrition facts per serving: calories 311, fat 13.5, fiber 6, carbs 18.0, protein 8

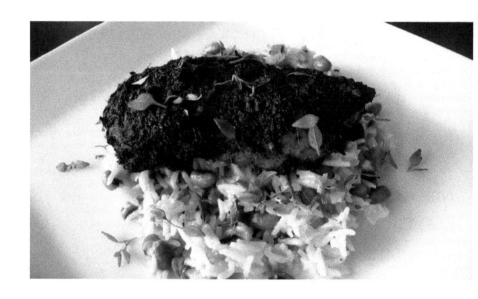

Chili and Fennel Bowls

Prep time: 5 minutes I**Cooking time:** 0 minutes I

Servings: 4

Ingredients:

- 2 spring onion, chopped
- 2 fennel bulbs, shredded
- 1 green chili pepper, chopped
- 1 tomato, chopped
- 1 teaspoon turmeric powder
- 1 teaspoon lime juice
- 2 tablespoons coriander, chopped
- Black pepper to the taste

Directions:

1. In a salad bowl, mix the fennel with the onions and the other ingredients, toss, divide into cups and serve.

Nutrition facts per serving: calories 310, fat 11.5, fiber 5.1, carbs 22.3, protein 6.5

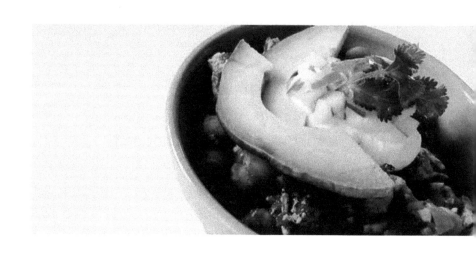

Sprouts Bites

Prep time: 10 minutes I **Cooking time:** 25 minutes I
Servings: 4

Ingredients:

- 1 pound Brussels sprouts, trimmed and halved
- 2 tablespoons olive oil
- 1 tablespoon cumin, ground
- 1 cup dill, chopped
- 2 garlic cloves, minced

Directions:

1. In a roasting pan, combine the Brussels sprouts with the oil and the other ingredients, toss and bake at 390 degrees F for 25 minutes.
2. Divide the sprouts into bowls and serve as a snack.

Nutrition facts per serving: calories 270, fat 10.3, fiber 5.2, carbs 11.1, protein 6

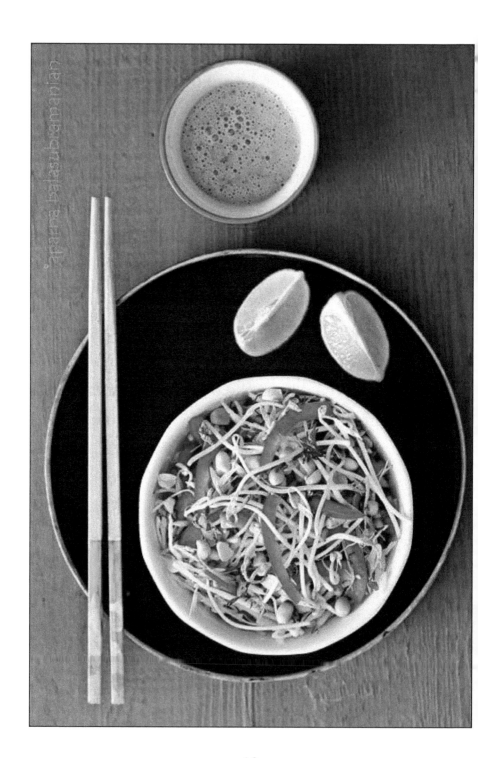

Walnuts Snack

Prep time: 10 minutes I **Cooking time:** 15 minutes I

Servings: 4

Ingredients:

- 2 cups walnuts
- 3 tablespoons red vinegar
- A drizzle of olive oil
- A pinch of cayenne pepper
- A pinch of red pepper flakes
- Black pepper to the taste

Directions:

1. Spread the walnuts on a lined baking sheet, add the vinegar and the other ingredients, toss, and roast at 400 degrees F for 15 minutes.
2. Divide the walnuts into bowls and serve.

Nutrition facts per serving: calories 280, fat 12.2, fiber 2, carbs 15.8, protein 6

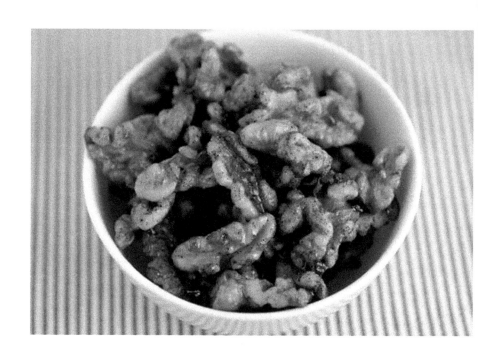

Radish Chips

Prep time: 10 minutes I **Cooking time:** 20 minutes I
Servings: 4

Ingredients:
- 1 pound radishes, thinly sliced
- A pinch of turmeric powder
- Black pepper for taste
- 2 tablespoons olive oil

Directions:
1. Spread the radish chips on a lined baking sheet, add the oil and the other ingredients, toss and bake at 400 degrees F for 20 minutes.
2. Divide the chips into bowls and serve.

Nutrition facts per serving: calories 120, fat 8.3, fiber 1, carbs 3.8, protein 6

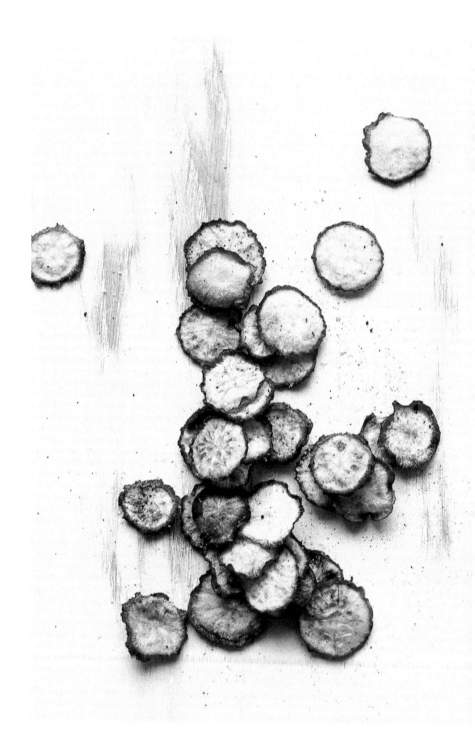

Leeks Bowls

Prep time: 4 minutes I **Cooking time:** 0 minutes I

Servings: 4

Ingredients:

- 4 leeks, sliced
- 1 cup cilantro, chopped
- Juice of 1 lime
- 1 tablespoon lime zest, grated
- 1 cup cherry tomatoes, halved
- 2 tablespoons olive oil
- Salt and black pepper to the taste

Directions:

1. In a salad bowl, mix the leeks and the other ingredients, toss, divide into small cups and serve.

Nutrition facts per serving: calories 280, fat 9.1, fiber 5.2, carbs 12.6, protein 5

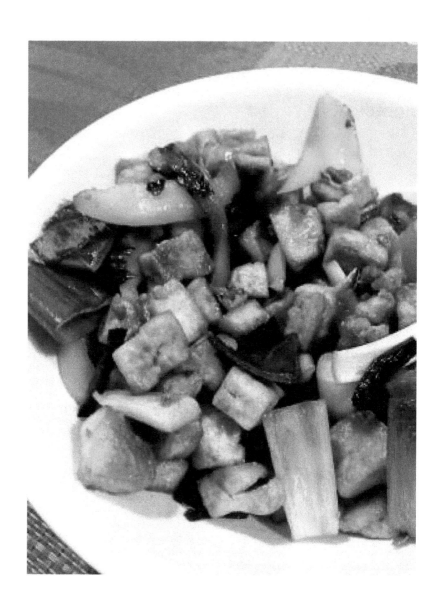

Creamy Leeks Dip

Prep time: 5 minutes I **Cooking time:** 0 minutes I
Servings: 4

Ingredients:
- 1 tablespoon lemon juice
- ½ cup cream cheese
- 2 tablespoons olive oil
- Black pepper to the taste
- 4 leeks, chopped
- 1 tablespoon cilantro, chopped

Directions:
1. In a blender, combine the cream cheese with the leeks and the other ingredients, pulse well, divide into bowls and serve as a party dip.

Nutrition facts per serving: calories 300, fat 12.2, fiber 7.6, carbs 14.7, protein 5.6

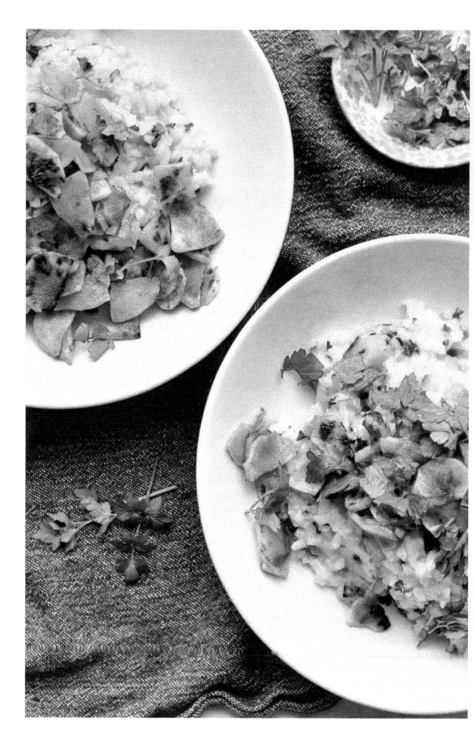

Peppers Cups

Prep time: 5 minutes I **Cooking time:** 0 minutes I
Servings: 4

Ingredients:

- ½ pound red bell pepper, cut into thin strips
- 3 green onions, chopped
- 1 tablespoon olive oil
- 2 teaspoons ginger, grated
- ½ teaspoon rosemary, dried
- 3 tablespoons balsamic vinegar

Directions:

1. In a salad bowl, mix the bell peppers with the onions and the other ingredients, toss, divide into small cups and serve.

Nutrition facts per serving: calories 160, fat 6, fiber 3, carbs 10.9, protein 5.2

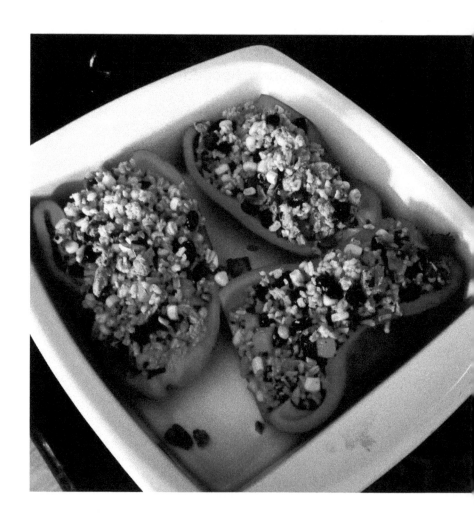

Coconut Avocado Spread

Prep time: 4 minutes I **Cooking time:** 0 minutes I

Servings: 4

Ingredients:

- 2 tablespoons dill, chopped
- 1 shallot, chopped
- 2 garlic cloves, minced
- 2 avocados, peeled, pitted and chopped
- 1 cup coconut cream
- 2 tablespoons olive oil
- 2 tablespoons lime juice
- Black pepper to the taste

Directions:

1. In a blender, combine the avocados with the shallots, garlic and the other ingredients, pulse well, divide into small bowls and serve as a snack.

Nutrition facts per serving: calories 300, fat 22.3, fiber 6.4, carbs 42, protein 8.9

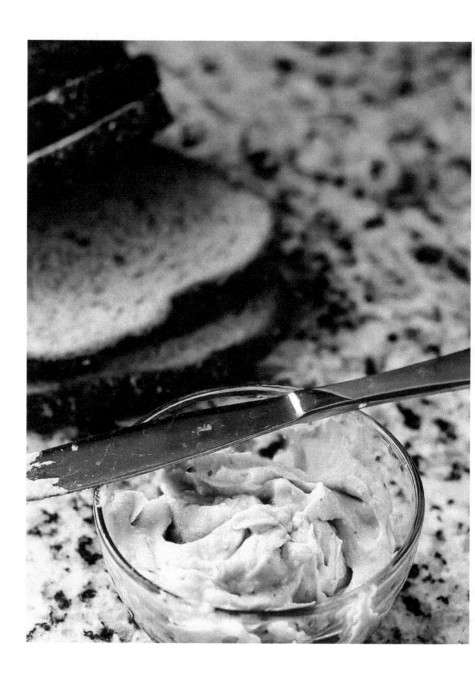

Lemon Corn Dip

Prep time: 30 minutes I **Cooking time:** 0 minutes I
Servings: 4

Ingredients:

- A pinch of cayenne pepper
- A pinch of black pepper
- 2 cups corn
- 1 cup coconut cream
- 2 tablespoons lemon juice
- 2 tablespoon avocado oil

Directions:

1. In a blender, combine the corn with the cream and the other ingredients, pulse well, divide into bowls and serve as a party dip.

Nutrition facts per serving: calories 215, fat 16.2, fiber 3.8, carbs 18.4, protein 4

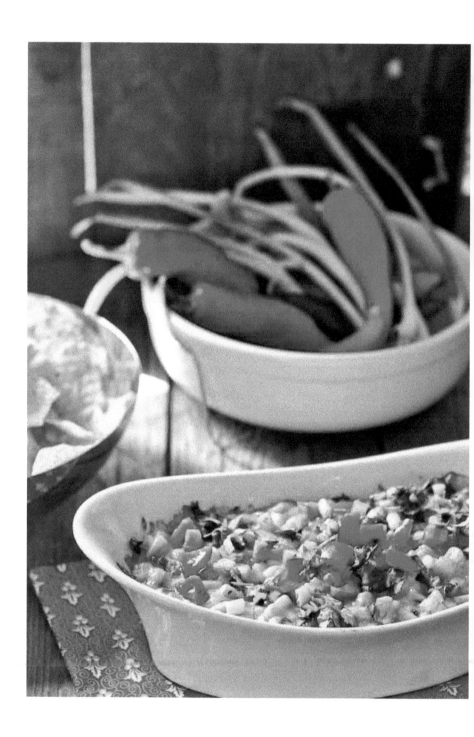

Beans and Chia Power Bars

Prep time: 2 hours I **Cooking time:** 0 minutes I

Servings: 12

Ingredients:

- 1 cup black beans, cooked
- 1 cup coconut flakes, unsweetened
- 1 cup butter
- ½ cup chia seeds
- ½ cup coconut cream

Directions:

1. In a blender, combine the beans with the coconut flakes and the other ingredients, pulse well, spread this into a square pan, press, keep in the fridge for 2 hours, slice into medium bars and serve.

Nutrition facts per serving: calories 141, fat 7, fiber 5, carbs 16.2, protein 5

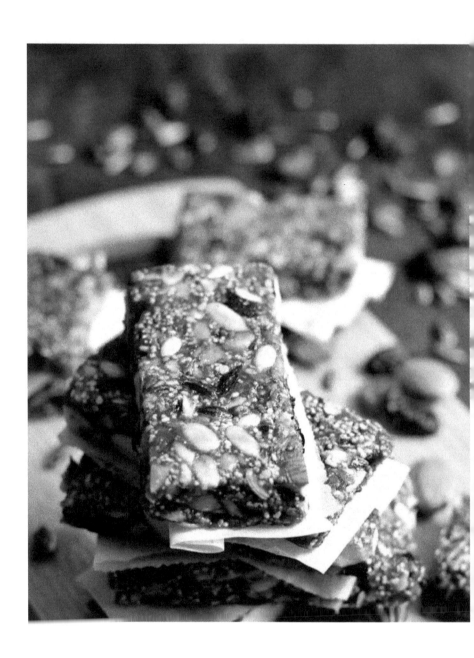

Apple Chips Mix

Prep time: 10 minutes I **Cooking time:** 2 hours I

Servings: 4

Ingredients:

- Cooking spray
- 2 teaspoons nutmeg, ground
- 1 cup pumpkin seeds
- 2 apples, cored and thinly sliced

Directions:

1. Arrange the pumpkin seeds and the apple chips on a lined baking sheet, sprinkle the nutmeg all over, grease them with the spray, introduce in the oven and bake at 300 degrees F for 2 hours.
2. Divide into bowls and serve as a snack.

Nutrition facts per serving: calories 80, fat 0, fiber 3, carbs 7, protein 4

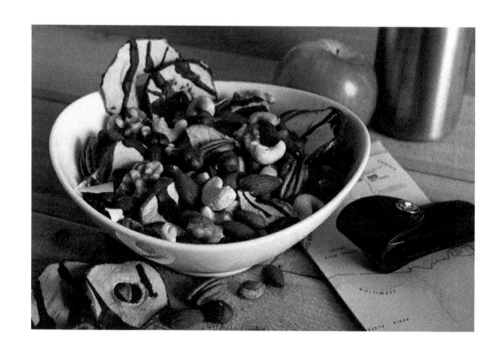

Yogurt Dip

Prep time: 5 minutes I **Cooking time:** 0 minutes I

Servings: 4

Ingredients:

- 2 cups Greek yogurt
- 1 tablespoon parsley, chopped
- ¼ cup tomatoes, chopped
- 2 tablespoons chives, chopped
- Black pepper to the taste

Directions:

1. In a bowl, mix the yogurt with the parsley and the other ingredients, whisk well, divide into small bowls and serve as a party dip.

Nutrition facts per serving: calories 78, fat 0, fiber 0.2, carbs 10.6, protein 8.2

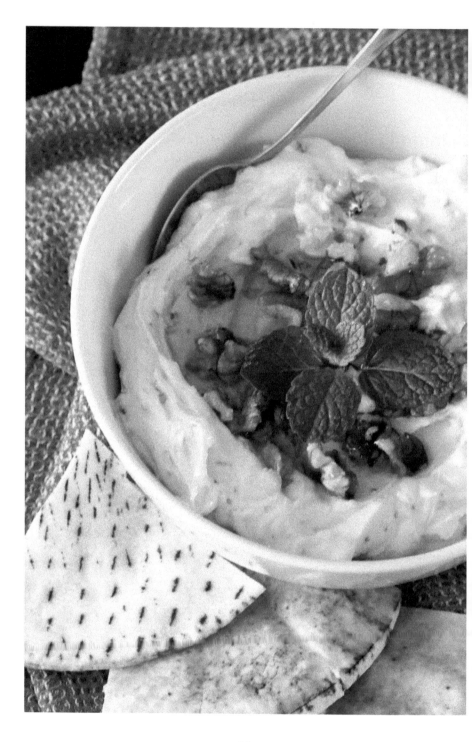

Beet Bites

Prep time: 10 minutes I **Cooking time:** 35 minutes I
Servings: 2

Ingredients:

- 1 teaspoon cayenne pepper
- 2 beets, peeled and cubed
- 1 teaspoon rosemary, dried
- 1 tablespoon olive oil
- 2 teaspoons lime juice

Directions:

1. In a roasting pan, combine the beet bites with the cayenne and the other ingredients, toss, introduce in the oven, roast at 355 degrees F for 35 minutes, divide into small bowls and serve as a snack.

Nutrition facts per serving: calories 170, fat 12.2, fiber 7, carbs 15.1, protein 6

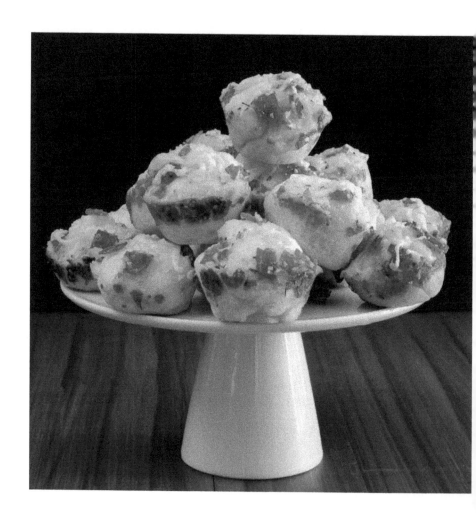

Pecans Bowls

Prep time: 10 minutes I **Cooking time:** 10 minutes I
Servings: 4

Ingredients:

- 2 cup walnuts
- 1 cup pecans, chopped
- 1 teaspoon avocado oil
- ½ teaspoon sweet paprika

Directions:

1. Spread the grapes and pecans on a lined baking sheet, add the oil and the paprika, toss, and bake at 400 degrees F for 10 minutes.
2. Divide into bowls and serve as a snack.

Nutrition facts per serving: calories 220, fat 12.4, fiber 3, carbs 12.9, protein 5.6

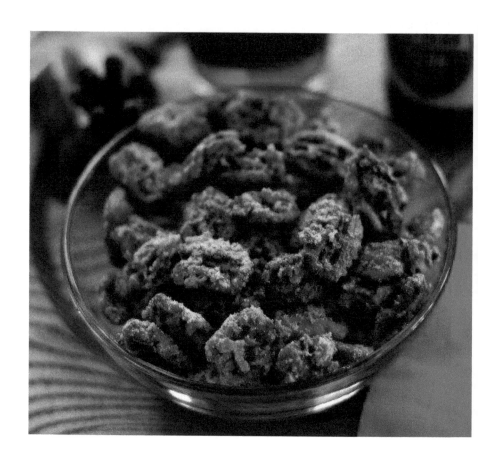

Salmon Muffins

Prep time: 10 minutes I **Cooking time:** 25 minutes I
Servings: 4

Ingredients:

- 1 cup mozzarella cheese, shredded
- 8 ounces smoked salmon, skinless, boneless, and chopped
- 1 cup almond flour
- 1 egg, whisked
- 1 teaspoon parsley, dried
- 1 garlic clove, minced
- Black pepper to the taste
- Cooking spray

Directions:

1. In a bowl, combine the salmon with the mozzarella and the other ingredients except the cooking spray and stir well.
2. Divide this mix into a muffin tray greased with the cooking spray, bake in the oven at 375 degrees F for 25 minutes and serve as a snack.

Nutrition facts per serving: calories 273, fat 17, fiber 3.5, carbs 6.9, protein 21.8

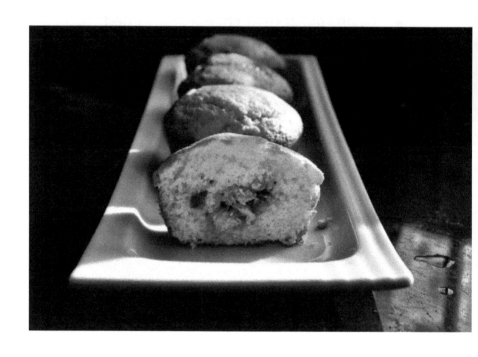

Squash Bites

Prep time: 10 minutes I **Cooking time:** 20 minutes I
Servings: 8

Ingredients:

- A drizzle of olive oil
- 1 big butternut squash, peeled and minced
- 2 tablespoons cilantro, chopped
- 2 eggs, whisked
- ½ cup whole wheat flour
- Black pepper to the taste
- 2 shallots, chopped
- 2 garlic cloves, minced

Directions:

1. In a bowl, mix the squash with the cilantro and the other ingredients except the oil, stir well and shape medium balls out of this mix.
2. Arrange them on a lined baking sheet, grease them with the oil, bake at 400 degrees F for 10 minutes on each side, divide into bowls and serve.

Nutrition facts per serving: calories 78, fat 3, fiber 0.9, carbs 10.8, protein 2.7

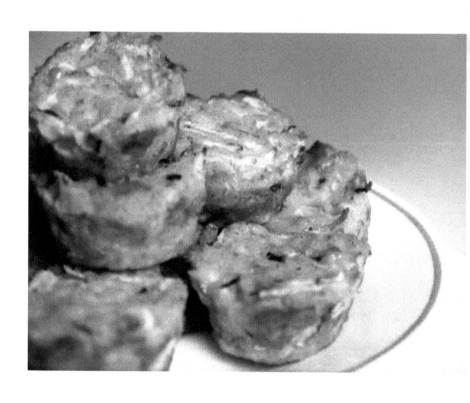

Green Beans Snack Bowls

Prep time: 10 minutes I **Cooking time:** 30 minutes I
Servings: 8

Ingredients:

- 1 pound green beans, trimmed
- 3 tablespoons parsley, chopped
- 1 tablespoon chives, chopped
- Black pepper to the taste
- 1 cup mozzarella, grated
- 1 tablespoon olive oil

Directions:

1. Spread the beans on a lined baking sheet, add the oil, parsley, chives and the black pepper and toss.
2. Sprinkle the mozzarella on top, bake at 390 degrees F for 30 minutes, divide into bowls and serve cold as a snack.

Nutrition facts per serving: calories 136, fat 2.7, fiber 6, carbs 25.9, protein 4.1

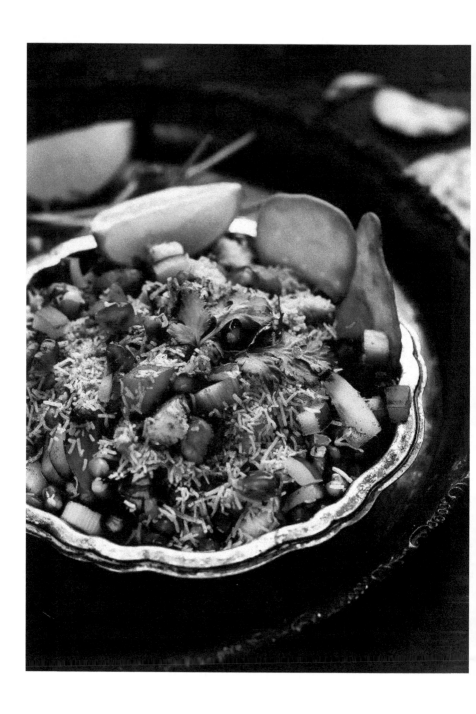

Broccoli and Shrimp Bars

Prep time: 10 minutes I **Cooking time:** 25 minutes I
Servings: 8

Ingredients:

- 1 pound broccoli florets, chopped
- ½ pound shrimp, peeled, deveined and chopped
- ½ cup mozzarella cheese, shredded
- 2 eggs, whisked
- 1 teaspoon oregano, dried
- 1 teaspoon basil, dried
- Black pepper to the taste

Directions:

1. In a bowl, mix the broccoli with the cheese and the other ingredients, stir well, spread into a rectangle pan and press well on the bottom.
2. Introduce in the oven at 380 degrees F, bake for 25 minutes, cut into bars and serve cold.

Nutrition facts per serving: calories 46, fat 1.3, fiber 1.8, carbs 4.2, protein 5

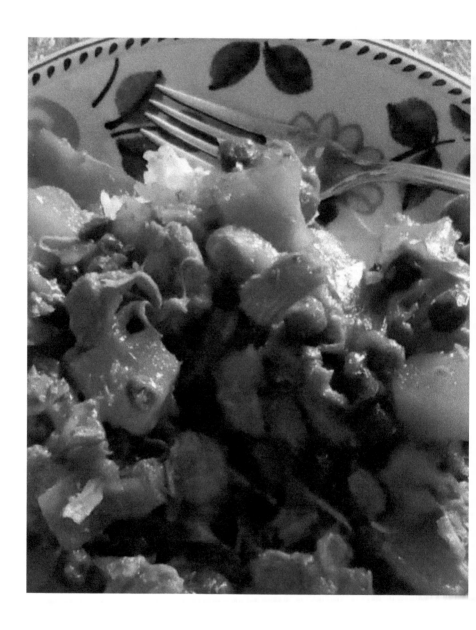

Pineapple and Basil Salsa

Prep time: 10 minutes I **Cooking time:** 40 minutes I
Servings: 4

Ingredients:

- 20 ounces pineapple, cubed
- 1 cup sun-dried tomatoes, cubed
- 3 tablespoons basil, chopped
- 1 tablespoon avocado oil
- 1 teaspoon lime juice
- 1 cup black olives, pitted and sliced
- Black pepper to the taste

Directions:

1. In a bowl, combine the pineapple cubes with the tomatoes and the other ingredients, toss, divide into smaller cups and serve as a snack.

Nutrition facts per serving: calories 125, fat 4.3, fiber 3.8, carbs 23.6, protein 1.5

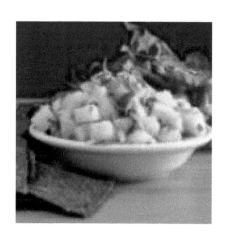

Lemon Pork Chops

Prep time: 10 minutes I **Cooking time:** 40 minutes I
Servings: 4

Ingredients:

- 1 pound pork chops
- 1 yellow onion, chopped
- 2 tablespoons olive oil
- ½ cup vegetable stock
- 2 tablespoons lemon juice
- A pinch of salt and black pepper
- 2 tablespoons chives, chopped

Directions:

1. In a roasting pan, combine the pork chops with the onion, the oil and the other ingredients, toss and bake at 390 degrees F for 40 minutes.
2. Divide the pork chops between plates and serve.

Nutrition info per serving: calories 439, fat 35.8, fiber 0.7, carbs 3.3, protein 25.9

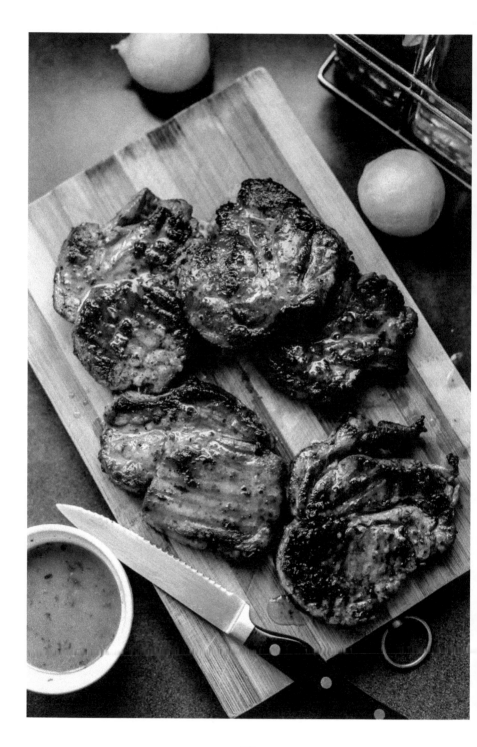

Lime Pork and Berries Mix

Prep time: 10 minutes I **Cooking time:** 35 minutes I
Servings: 4

Ingredients:

- 4 pork chops
- 2 tablespoons olive oil
- 1 teaspoon chili powder
- 1 teaspoon rosemary, dried
- 1 cup blueberries
- 1 tablespoon lime juice
- A pinch of salt and black pepper
- ½ teaspoon thyme, dried
- 1 tablespoon balsamic vinegar
- A pinch of salt and black pepper

Directions:

1. Heat up a pan with the oil over medium heat, add the pork chops and brown for 2 minutes on each side.
2. Add the rest of the ingredients, toss, cook over medium heat for 30 minutes more, divide between plates and serve.

Nutrition info per serving: calories 344, fat 27.2, fiber 1.4, carbs 6.9, protein 18.4

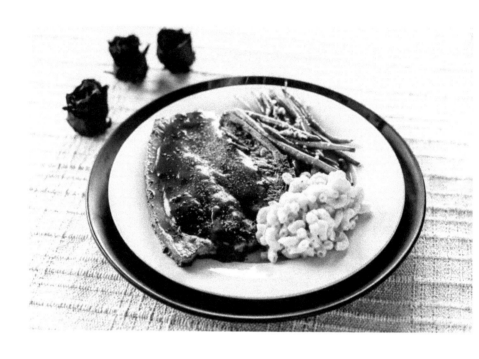

Cilantro Pork

Prep time: 10 minutes I **Cooking time:** 30 minutes I
Servings: 4

Ingredients:

- 4 pork chops
- 2 tablespoons coconut aminos
- 2 tablespoons olive oil
- A pinch of salt and black pepper
- 1 tablespoon cinnamon powder
- ½ teaspoon cumin, ground
- 1 tablespoon cilantro, chopped

Directions:

1. Heat up a pan with the oil over medium heat, add the pork chops and cook for 2 minutes on each side.
2. Add the rest of the ingredients, toss, introduce in the oven and bake at 390 degrees F for 25 minutes more.
3. Divide everything between plates and serve.

Nutrition info per serving: calories 317, fat 26.9, fiber 0.1, carbs 0.2, protein 18

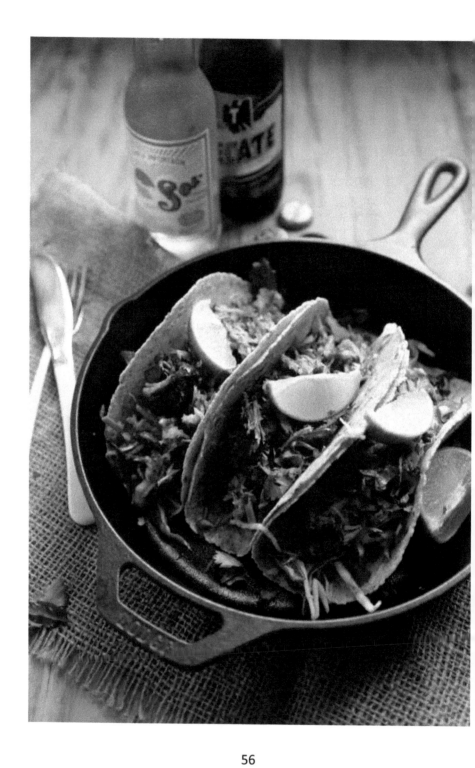

Pepper Chops

Prep time: 10 minutes I **Cooking time:** 35 minutes I

Servings: 4

Ingredients:

- 4 pork chops
- 1 yellow onion, chopped
- 2 tablespoons olive oil
- Juice of 2 lemons
- 1 teaspoon red pepper, crushed
- A pinch of salt and black pepper
- 1 tablespoon cilantro, chopped

Directions:

1. In a roasting pan, combine the pork chops with the onion, the oil and the other ingredients, toss and bake at 390 degrees F for 35 minutes.
2. Divide the pork chops between plates and serve with a side salad.

Nutrition info per serving: calories 339, fat 27.1, fiber 1.1, carbs 5.1, protein 18.7

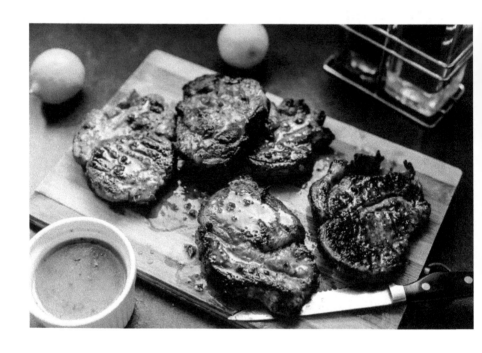

Herbed Pork

Prep time: 10 minutes I **Cooking time:** 45 minutes I
Servings: 4

Ingredients:

- 2 pounds pork stew meat, cubed
- 2 sweet potatoes, peeled and cut into wedges
- 2 tablespoons olive oil
- 1 teaspoon chili powder
- 1 teaspoon black peppercorns, crushed
- Juice of 1 lemon
- 3 garlic cloves, minced
- 1 tablespoon thyme, chopped
- 1 tablespoon basil, chopped
- ½ tablespoon oregano, chopped
- ½ tablespoon rosemary, chopped

Directions:

1. In a roasting pan, combine the meat with the potatoes, the oil, chili powder and the other ingredients, toss and bake at 390 degrees F for 45 minutes.
2. Divide everything between plates and serve.

Nutrition info per serving: calories 251, fat 5, fiber 9, carbs 15, protein 7

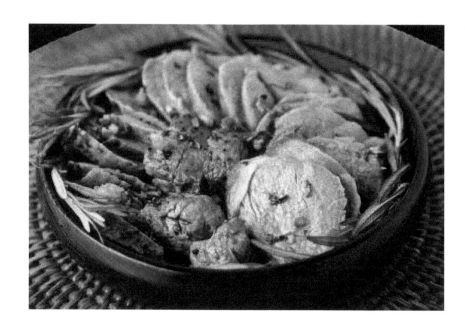

Paprika Pork and Scallions

Prep time: 10 minutes I **Cooking time:** 30 minutes I

Servings: 4

Ingredients:

- 4 scallions, chopped
- 2 garlic cloves, minced
- 2 tablespoons olive oil
- 2 pounds pork stew meat, cubed
- 1 teaspoon sweet paprika
- A pinch of salt and black pepper
- ½ cup mustard
- 1 tablespoon chives, chopped

Directions:

1. Heat up a pan with the oil over medium heat, add the scallions and the garlic and sauté for 5 minutes.
2. Add the meat and brown it for 5 minutes.
3. Add the rest of the ingredients, toss, cook over medium heat for 20 minutes more, divide into bowls and serve.

Nutrition info per serving: calories 271, fat 5, fiber 6, carbs 15, protein 20

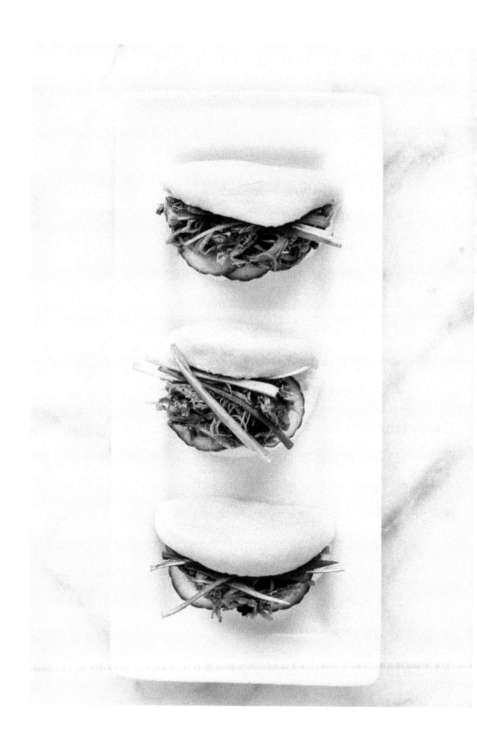

Cumin Pork Chops

Prep time: 10 minutes I **Cooking time:** 30 minutes I
Servings: 4

Ingredients:

- 4 pork chops
- 4 garlic cloves, minced
- 2 tablespoons olive oil
- 1 cup vegetable stock
- 1 teaspoon rosemary, dried
- ½ teaspoon cumin, ground
- 2 tablespoons lemon juice
- A pinch of salt and black pepper

Directions:

1. Heat up a pan with the oil over medium heat, add the garlic and sauté it for 2 minutes.
2. Add the meat and brown it for 5 minutes more.
3. Add the remaining ingredients, toss, bring to a simmer and cook over medium heat for 23 minutes more.
4. Divide the mix between plates and serve.

Nutrition info per serving: calories 261, fat 6, fiber 7, carbs 15, protein 16

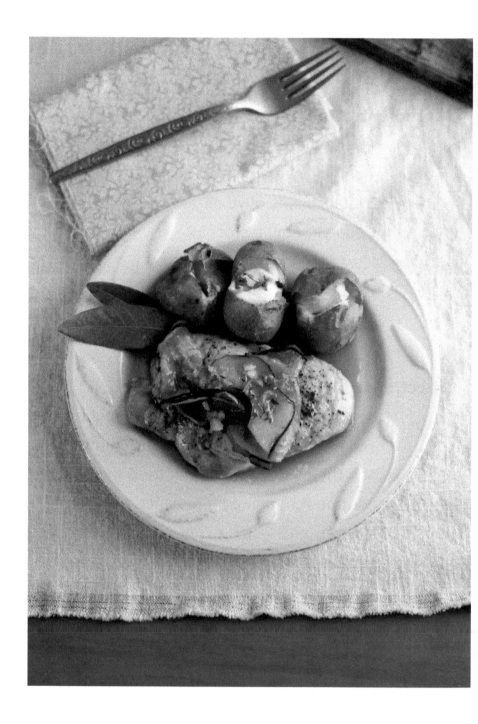

Spiced Pork Mix

Prep time: 10 minutes I **Cooking time:** 35 minutes I
Servings: 4

Ingredients:

- 4 pork chops
- 1 yellow onion, chopped
- 2 tablespoons olive oil
- 1/3 cup walnuts, chopped
- ½ teaspoon turmeric powder
- ½ teaspoon coriander, ground
- 2 teaspoons garlic powder
- A pinch of salt and black pepper
- 1 teaspoon smoked paprika
- 1 teaspoon chipotle chili powder
- ¼ cup vegetable stock
- 1 tablespoon cilantro, chopped

Directions:

1. Heat up a pan with the oil over medium heat, add the onion and the meat and brown for 5 minutes.
2. Add the turmeric, coriander, the walnuts and the other ingredients, toss, cook over medium heat for 30 minutes more.
3. Divide everything between plates and serve.

Nutrition info per serving: calories 251, fat 12, fiber 4, carbs 7, protein 16

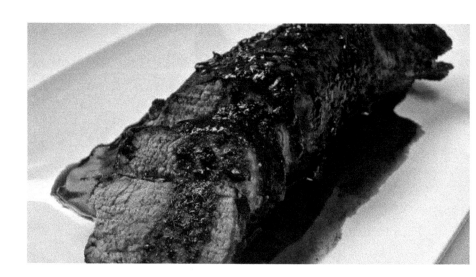

Pork and Asparagus

Prep time: 10 minutes I **Cooking time:** 40 minutes I
Servings: 4

Ingredients:
- 1 pound pork chops
- 2 tablespoons olive oil
- 1 bunch asparagus, trimmed and halved
- 1 teaspoon sweet paprika
- A pinch of salt and black pepper
- 4 garlic cloves, minced
- ½ cup veggie stock

Directions:
1. Heat up a pan with the oil over medium-high heat, add the pork chops and brown for 5 minutes.
2. Add the rest of the ingredients, toss, introduce the pan in the oven and bake at 380 degrees F for 35 minutes.
3. Divide everything between plates and serve.

Nutrition info per serving: calories 282, fat 12, fiber 1, carbs 6, protein 17

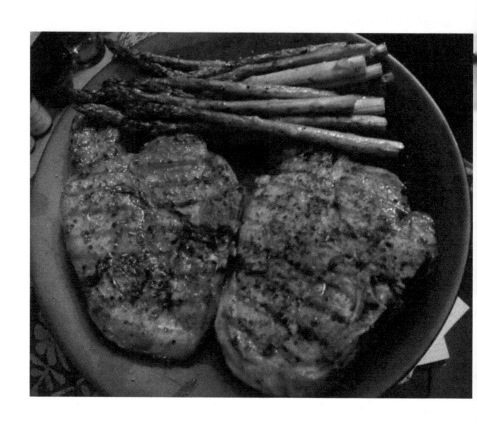

Pork and Black Beans

Prep time: 10 minutes I **Cooking time:** 35 minutes I

Servings: 4

Ingredients:

- 2 pounds pork stew meat, cubed
- 1 yellow onion, chopped
- 1 cup black beans, cooked
- 3 tablespoons olive oil
- A pinch of salt and black pepper
- 1 teaspoon cumin, ground
- ¼ teaspoon coriander, ground

Directions:

1. Heat up a pan with the oil over medium-high heat, add the onion and sauté for 5 minutes.
2. Add the meat and brown for 5 minutes more.
3. Add the rest of the ingredients, bring to a simmer and cook over medium heat for 25 minutes.
4. Divide everything between plates and serve.

Nutrition info per serving: calories 261, fat 6, fiber 5, carbs 11, protein 18

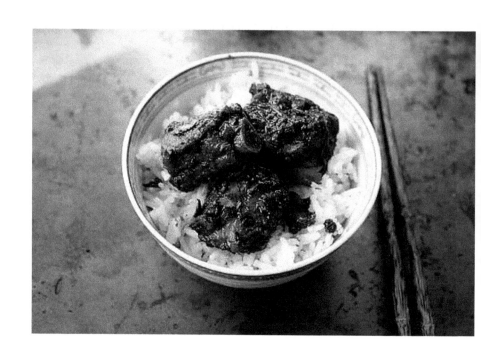

Peppercorn Pork Mix

Prep time: 10 minutes I **Cooking time:** 8 hours I
Servings: 4

Ingredients:

- 2 pounds pork stew meat, cubed
- 1 yellow onion, sliced
- 1 cup blackberries
- ½ teaspoon rosemary, dried
- ½ teaspoon black peppercorns, crushed
- A pinch of salt and black pepper
- Juice of ½ lemon
- 2 garlic cloves, minced

Directions:

1. In your slow cooker, mix the pork with the onion, the berries and the other ingredients, toss, put the lid on and cook on Low for 8 hours.
2. Divide everything between plates and serve.

Nutrition Info per serving: calories 261, fat 4, fiber 8, carbs 9, protein 17

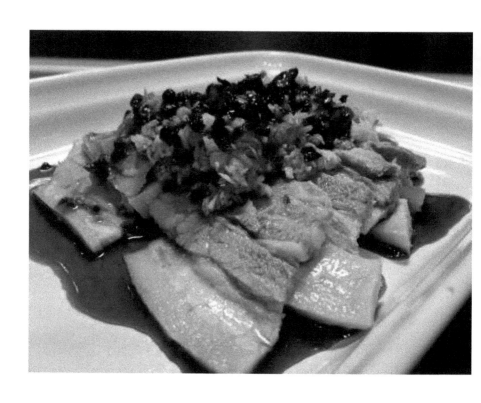

Balsamic Oregano Pork

Prep time: 10 minutes I **Cooking time:** 40 minutes I
Servings: 4

Ingredients:

- 4 pork chops
- 1 yellow onion, chopped
- 2 tablespoons avocado oil
- ¼ cup lime juice
- 4 garlic cloves, minced
- 1 tablespoon chili powder
- ½ teaspoon red pepper, crushed
- 2 tablespoons balsamic vinegar
- 1 teaspoon oregano, dried
- 1 teaspoon cloves
- 2 tablespoons cilantro, chopped

Directions:

1. Heat up a pan with the oil over medium heat, add the onion and the garlic and sauté for 5 minutes.
2. Add the meat and brown for 5 more minutes.
3. Add the rest of the ingredients, toss, cook over medium heat for 30 minutes, divide everything between plates and serve.

Nutrition info per serving: calories 271, fat 7, fiber 5, carbs 11, protein 16

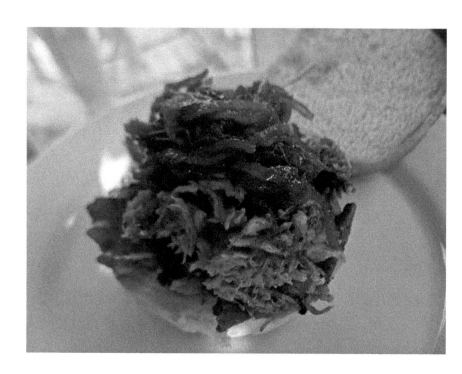

Sage Pork Mix

Prep time: 10 minutes I **Cooking time:** 40 minutes I
Servings: 4

Ingredients:

- 1 pound pork stew meat, roughly cubed
- 1 yellow onion, chopped
- 2 tablespoons avocado oil
- A pinch of salt and black pepper
- ½ cup vegetable stock
- 2 garlic cloves, minced
- 2 cups Brussels sprouts, trimmed and halved
- 1 tablespoon sage, chopped

Directions:

1. Heat up a pan with the oil over medium-high heat, add the onion and the garlic and sauté for 5 minutes.
2. Add the meat and brown for 5 minutes more.
3. Add the remaining ingredients, toss, and bake at 390 degrees F for 30 minutes.
4. Divide the mix between plates and serve.

Nutrition info per serving: calories 251, fat 6, fiber 8, carbs 12, protein 17

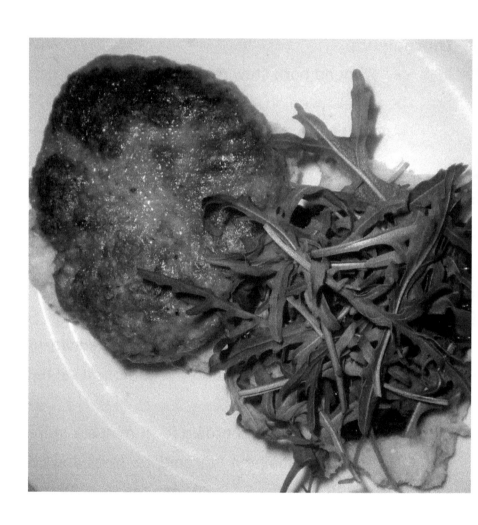

Pork Chops and Tomato Sauce

Prep time: 5 minutes I **Cooking time:** 1 hour I
Servings: 4

Ingredients:

- 2 tablespoons olive oil
- 2 pounds pork chops
- 4 scallions, chopped
- A pinch of salt and black pepper
- 2 garlic cloves, minced
- ¼ cup chicken stock
- 1 cup tomato sauce
- 2 tablespoons lime juice
- 1 tablespoon herbs de Provence

Directions:

1. Heat up a pan with the oil over medium heat, add the scallions and the garlic and sauté for 5 minutes.
2. Add the meat and brown for 5 minutes more.
3. Add the remaining ingredients, toss and bake everything at 380 degrees F for 50 minutes.
4. Divide the whole mix between plates and serve.

Nutrition info per serving: calories 251, fat 3, fiber 6, carbs 9, protein 16

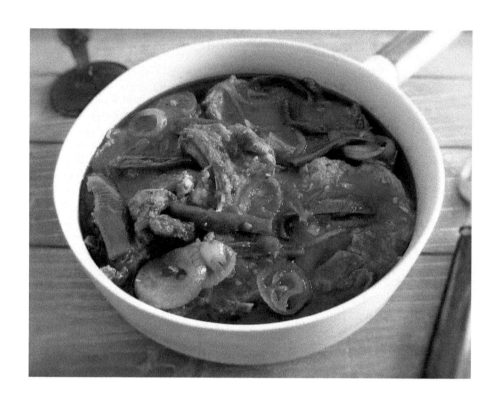

Pork Chops and Citrus Sauce

Prep time: 10 minutes I **Cooking time:** 50 minutes I

Servings: 4

Ingredients:

- 4 pork chops
- 4 spring onions, chopped
- 1 cup orange sauce
- 1 teaspoon turmeric powder
- 1 tablespoon olive oil
- 1 tablespoon chives, chopped
- A pinch of salt and black pepper

Directions:

1. Heat up a pan with the oil over medium-high heat, add the meat and brown for 5 minutes.
2. Add the spring onions and the other ingredients, toss, and bake at 390 degrees F for 45 minutes.
3. Divide everything between plates and serve.

Nutrition info per serving: calories 271, fat 5, fiber 8, carbs 10, protein 17

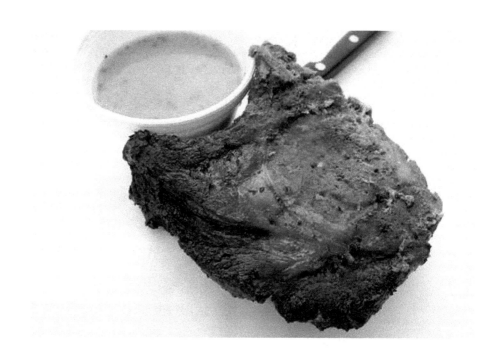

Allspice Pork

Prep time: 10 minutes I **Cooking time:** 1 hour I

Servings: 4

Ingredients:

- 2 tablespoons olive oil
- 2 pounds pork stew meat, cubed
- 1 teaspoon cumin, ground
- 1 tablespoon sage, chopped
- 1 yellow onion, chopped
- 1 cup vegetable stock
- A pinch of salt and black pepper
- 1 teaspoon chili pepper flakes, dried
- ½ teaspoon allspice, ground

Directions:

1. Heat up a pan with the oil over medium-high heat, add the onion and the meat and brown for 10 minutes.
2. Add the rest of the ingredients, toss, introduce in the oven and bake at 390 degrees F for 50 minutes.
3. Divide everything between plates and serve.

Nutrition info per serving: calories 261, fat 4, fiber 7, carbs 12, protein 18

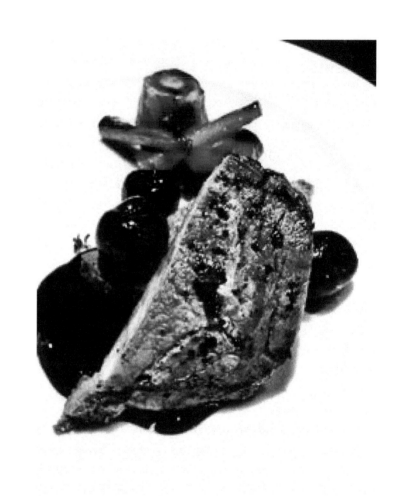

Pork with Mushrooms

Prep time: 10 minutes I **Cooking time:** 8 hours and 10 minutes I **Servings:** 4

Ingredients:

- 1 green bell pepper, chopped
- 1 red bell pepper, chopped
- 1 cup white mushrooms, sliced
- 1 pound pork stew meat, cubed
- 1 yellow onion, chopped
- 2 tablespoons olive oil
- Salt and black pepper to the taste
- 1 cup tomatoes, chopped
- 1 tablespoon parsley, chopped
- 2 teaspoons chili powder

Directions:

1. Heat up a pan with the oil over medium heat, add the onion and the mushrooms and sauté for 5 minutes.
2. Add the meat and brown for 5 minutes more.
3. Transfer everything to your slow cooker, add the rest of the ingredients, toss, put the lid on and cook on Low for 8 hours.
4. Divide everything between plates and serve.

Nutrition info per serving: calories 274, fat 6, fiber 3, carbs 11, protein 24

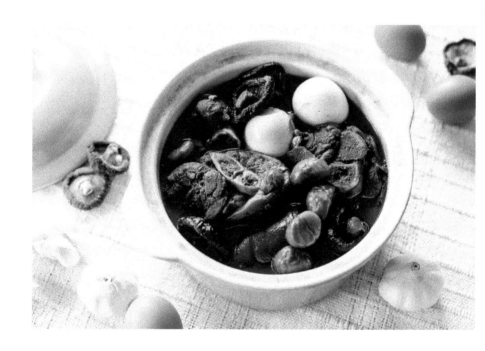

Chili Cinnamon Pork Mix

Prep time: 10 minutes I **Cooking time:** 1 hour I

Servings: 4

Ingredients:

- 2 pounds pork stew meat, cubed
- 2 tablespoons olive oil
- 1 yellow onion, chopped
- 2 avocados, peeled, pitted and sliced
- 1 tablespoon chili powder
- Salt and black pepper to the taste
- 1 teaspoon cumin, ground
- ½ teaspoon cinnamon powder
- A pinch of cayenne pepper
- ½ cup vegetable stock
- ½ cup parsley, chopped

Directions:

1. Heat up a pan with the oil over medium-high heat, add the onion and the meat and brown for 10 minutes stirring often.
2. Add the avocados and the other ingredients, toss, introduce the pan in the oven and bake at 390 degrees F for 50 minutes.
3. Divide the mix between plates and serve.

Nutrition info per serving: calories 300, fat 7, fiber 6, carbs 12, protein 18

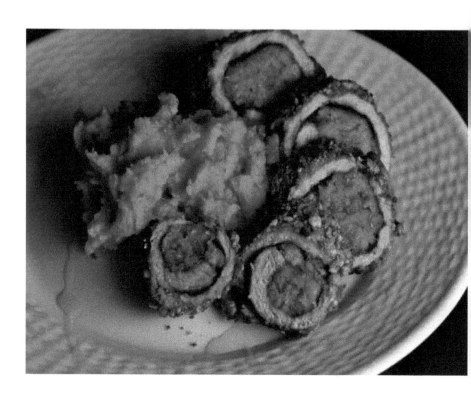

Pork with Cabbage

Prep time: 10 minutes I **Cooking time:** 45 minutes I
Servings: 4

Ingredients:

- 1 cup red cabbage, shredded
- 2 pounds pork stew meat, cubed
- 2 tablespoons olive oil
- 4 scallions, chopped
- 1 tablespoon balsamic vinegar
- A pinch of salt and black pepper
- 1 tablespoon cilantro, chopped

Directions:

1. Heat up a pan with the oil over medium-high heat, add the scallions and the meat and brown for 10 minutes.
2. Add the other ingredients, toss and cook over medium heat for 35 minutes.
3. Divide everything between plates and serve.

Nutrition info per serving: calories 260, fat 5, fiber 4, carbs 12, protein 14

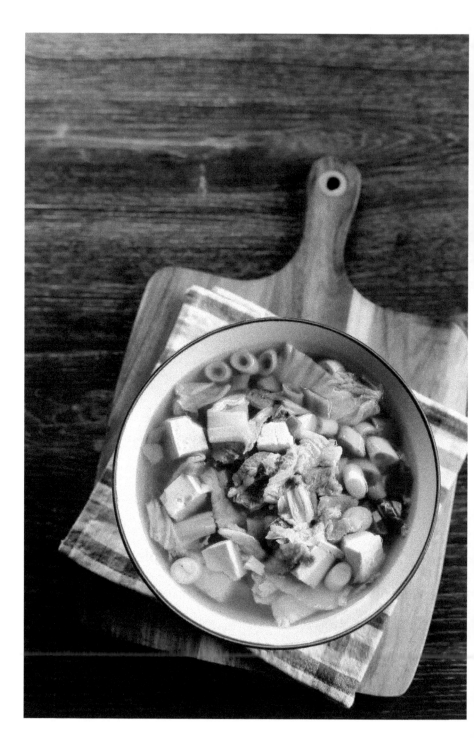

Pork with Scallions and Cauliflower

Prep time: 10 minutes I **Cooking time:** 8 hours I
Servings: 4

Ingredients:

- 2 pounds pork roast, sliced
- 4 scallions, chopped
- 2 garlic cloves, minced
- 1 yellow onion, chopped
- 2 tablespoons olive oil
- 1 cup cauliflower florets
- ½ cup vegetable stock
- A pinch of salt and black pepper
- A pinch of red chili pepper flakes

Directions:

1. In your slow cooker, mix the pork roast with the scallions, the garlic and the other ingredients, toss, put the lid on and cook on Low for 8 hours.
2. Divide everything between plates and serve.

Nutrition info per serving: calories 556, fat 29, fiber 1.7, carbs 6, protein 65.8

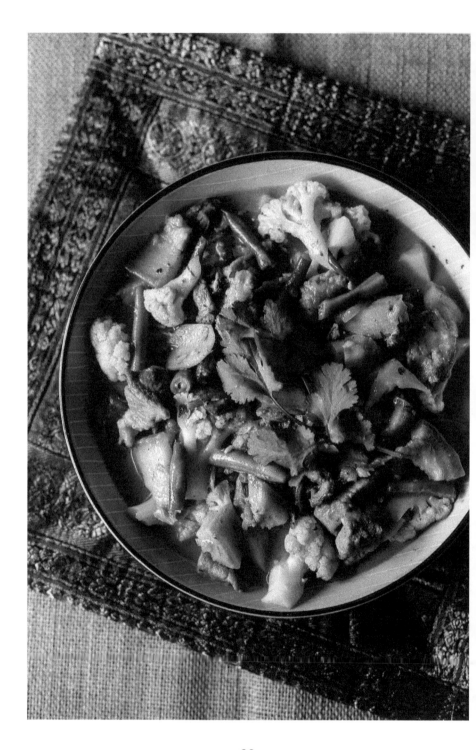

Paprika Pork with Grapes

Prep time: 10 minutes I **Cooking time:** 40 minutes I

Servings: 6

Ingredients:

- 2 pounds pork stew meat, cubed
- 2 spring onions, chopped
- 1 cup grapes, halved
- 2 tablespoons olive oil
- ¼ teaspoon coriander, ground
- ¼ teaspoon smoked paprika
- ¼ cup coconut aminos
- A pinch of salt and black pepper

Directions:

1. Heat up a pan with the oil over medium heat, add the onions and the meat and brown for 10 minutes.
2. Add the rest of the ingredients, toss, cook over medium heat for 30 minutes more, divide between plates and serve.

Nutrition info per serving: calories 574, fat 29, fiber 0.5, carbs 7.6, protein 66.7

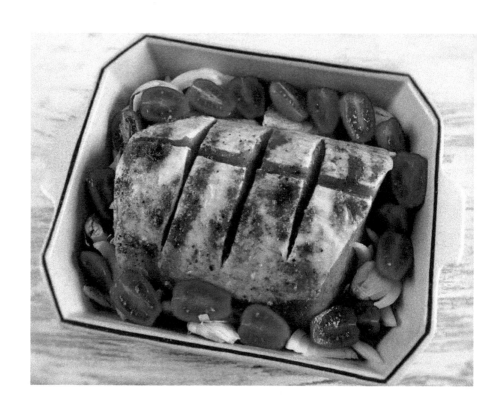

Pork with Kale

Prep time: 10 minutes I **Cooking time:** 50 minutes I
Servings: 4

Ingredients:

- 2 pound pork roast, sliced
- 2 tablespoons olive oil
- 4 scallions, chopped
- 2 green apples, cored and cut into wedges
- 1 cup baby kale
- A pinch of salt and black pepper
- 1 teaspoon chili powder
- 1 tablespoon thyme, chopped

Directions:

1. In a roasting pan, combine the roast with the oil, the apples and the other ingredients, toss and bake at 390 degrees F for 50 minutes.
2. Divide everything between plates and serve.

Nutrition info per serving: calories 605, fat 28.8, fiber 3.8, carbs 19.1, protein 65.9

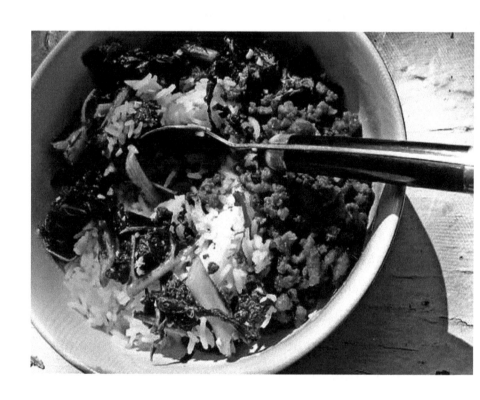

Balsamic Pork

Prep time: 10 minutes I **Cooking time:** 1 hour I
Servings: 4

Ingredients:

- 2 pounds pork stew meat, cubed
- 2 tablespoons olive oil
- ½ cup vegetable stock
- 1 yellow onion, chopped
- 1 tablespoon ginger, grated
- 2 tablespoons balsamic vinegar
- A pinch of salt and black pepper
- ½ teaspoon chili powder

Directions:

1. Heat up a pan with the oil over medium heat, add the onion and the ginger and sauté for 5 minutes.
2. Add the meat and other ingredients, toss, cook over medium heat for 45 minutes more, divide between plates and serve.

Nutrition info per serving: calories 280, fat 7.8, fiber 8, carbs 12, protein 15.6

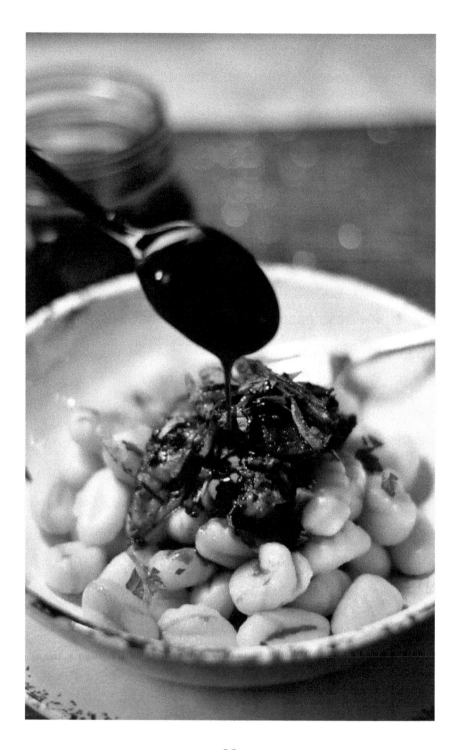

Cumin Pork and Mango Mix

Prep time: 10 minutes I **Cooking time:** 40 minutes I

Servings: 4

Ingredients:

- 2 pounds pork stew meat, cubed
- 4 scallions, chopped
- 1 tablespoon olive oil
- 1 teaspoon garlic powder
- 1 teaspoon cumin, ground
- 1 mango, peeled, pitted and cubed
- A pinch of salt and black pepper
- Juice of 1 lime
- ¼ cup cilantro, chopped

Directions:

1. Heat up a pan with the oil over medium heat, add the scallions and the meat and brown for 5 minutes.
2. Add the garlic powder, cumin and the other ingredients, toss, cook over medium heat for 35 minutes more, divide between plates and serve.

Nutrition info per serving: calories 200, fat 6, fiber 7, carbs 12, protein 16

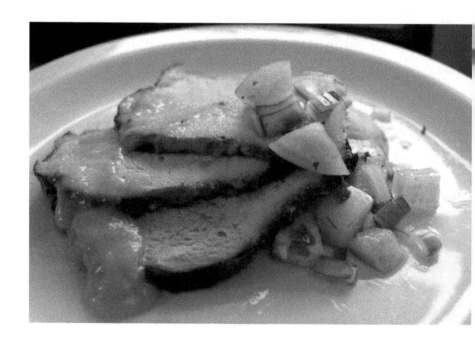

Pork and Pine Nuts Mix

Prep time: 10 minutes I **Cooking time:** 45 minutes I

Servings: 4

Ingredients:

- 2 pounds pork roast, sliced
- ¼ cup basil, chopped
- 1 tablespoon pine nuts, toasted
- 1 tablespoons garlic, minced
- 2 tablespoons olive oil
- ¼ cup vegetable stock
- A pinch of salt and black pepper
- 1 teaspoon coriander, ground
- 1 teaspoon onion powder

Directions:

1. In a blender, combine the basil with the pine nuts and the other ingredients except the roast and the stock and pulse well.
2. Put the roast slices on a baking dish, add the stock and the basil mix, toss and bake at 390 degrees F for 45 minutes.
3. Divide everything between plates and serve.

Nutrition info per serving: calories 270, fat 6, fiber 5, carbs 13, protein 18

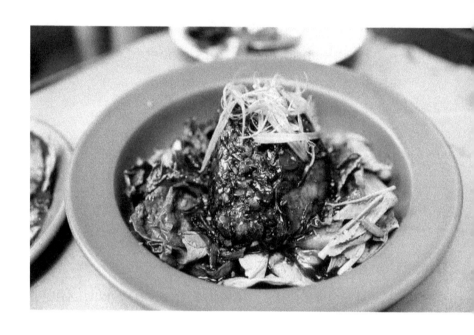

Pork with Tomatoes and Endives

Prep time: 10 minutes I **Cooking time:** 40 minutes I

Servings: 4

Ingredients:

- 2 green onions, chopped
- 2 pounds pork stew meat, roughly cubed
- 2 endives, shredded
- 4 garlic cloves, minced
- 1 cup cherry tomatoes, cubed
- A pinch of salt and black pepper
- ¾ cup coconut cream

Directions:

1. In a roasting pan, combine the pork meat with the endives and the other ingredients, toss and cook at 390 degrees F for 40 minutes.
2. Divide everything between plates and serve.

Nutrition info per serving: calories 261, fat 11, fiber 1, carbs 8, protein 18

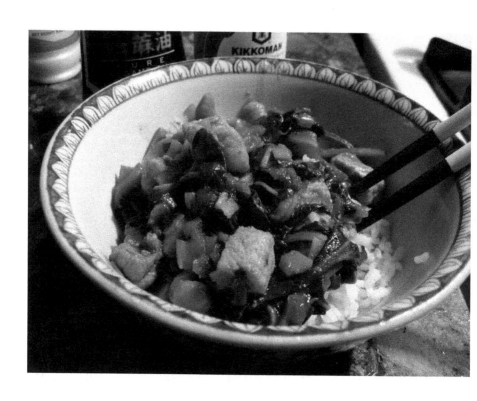

Pork and Shallots Pan

Prep time: 10 minutes I **Cooking time:** 40 minutes I

Servings: 4

Ingredients:

- 1 cup shallots, chopped
- ½ cup vegetable stock
- 2 pounds pork stew meat, roughly cubed
- 2 garlic cloves, minced
- A pinch of salt and black pepper
- 2 tablespoons olive oil
- 1 tablespoon cilantro, chopped

Directions:

1. Heat up a pan with the oil over medium-high heat, add the shallots and sauté for 10 minutes.
2. Add the meat and the other ingredients, toss, cook over medium heat for 30 minutes, divide between plates and serve.

Nutrition info per serving: calories 250, fat 12, fiber 2, carbs 13, protein 17

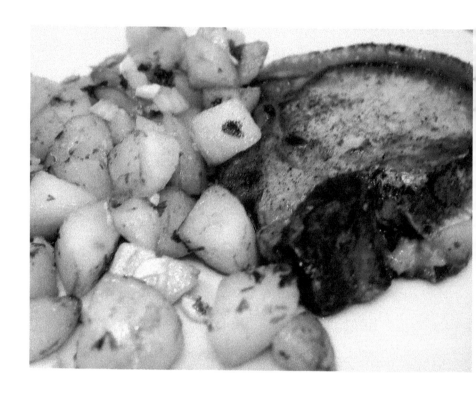

Mint Pork and Almonds

Prep time: 10 minutes I **Cooking time:** 40 minutes I

Servings: 4

Ingredients:

- 4 pork chops
- 1 cup mint leaves
- 2 tablespoons balsamic vinegar
- 1 tablespoon almonds, chopped
- 2 tablespoons olive oil
- 2 garlic cloves, minced
- Salt and black pepper to the taste
- ¼ teaspoon red pepper flakes

Directions:

1. In a blender, combine the mint with the vinegar and the other ingredients except the pork chops and pulse well.
2. Heat up a pan with the mint mix over medium heat, add the pork chops, toss, introduce in the oven and bake at 390 degrees F for 40 minutes.
3. Divide everything between plates and serve.

Nutrition info per serving: calories 260, fat 6 fiber 1, carbs 8, protein 23

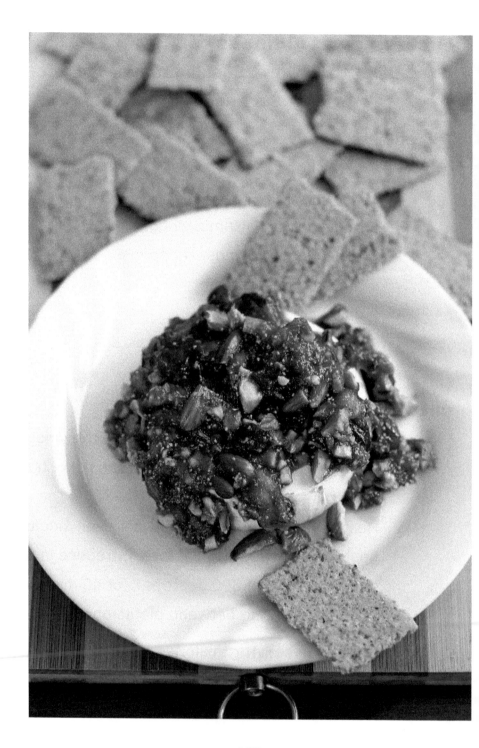

Pork and Zucchinis

Prep time: 10 minutes I **Cooking time:** 40 minutes I
Servings: 4

Ingredients:

- 2 pounds pork stew meat, roughly cubed
- 2 zucchinis, sliced
- 2 tablespoons olive oil
- 1 teaspoon nutmeg, ground
- 1 teaspoon cinnamon powder
- 1 teaspoon cumin, ground
- 2 tablespoons lime juice
- 2 garlic cloves, minced
- A pinch of sea salt and black pepper

Directions:

1. In a roasting pan, combine the meat with the zucchinis, the nutmeg and the other ingredients, toss and bake at 390 degrees F for 40 minutes.
2. Divide everything between plates and serve.

Nutrition info per serving: calories 200, fat 5, fiber 2, carbs 10, protein 22

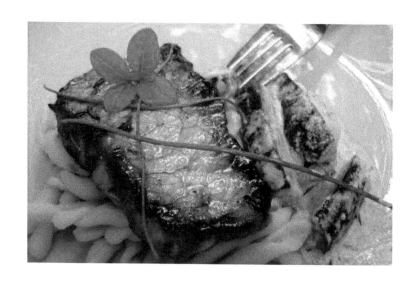

Pork and Pinto Beans

Prep time: 10 minutes I **Cooking time:** 1 hour I

Servings: 4

Ingredients:

- 2 pounds pork stew meat, roughly cubed
- 1 cup pinto beans, cooked
- 4 scallions, chopped
- 2 tablespoons olive oil
- 1 tablespoon chili powder
- 2 teaspoons cumin, ground
- A pinch of sea salt and black pepper
- 2 garlic cloves, minced
- 1 cup vegetable stock
- A handful parsley, chopped

Directions:

1. Heat up a pan with the oil over medium-high heat, add the scallions and the garlic and sauté for 5 minutes.
2. Add the meat and brown for 5 minutes more.
3. Add the beans and the other ingredients, toss, introduce the pan in the oven and cook everything at 380 degrees F for 50 minutes.
4. Divide the mix between plates and serve.

Nutrition info per serving: calories 291, fat 4, fiber 10, carbs 15, protein 24

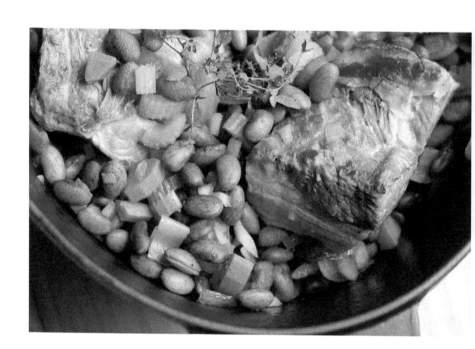

Lightning Source UK Ltd.
Milton Keynes UK
UKHW020803110621
385329UK00001B/106

9 781803 170671